AIP (AUTOIMMUNE PROTOCOL) DIET

Overview, Food List, and Guide

Nettie H. Crisler

CHAPTER 1

Autoimmune protocol(AIP) Diet

The Autoimmune protocol(AIP) is a diet regimen that goals to minimize swelling, discomfort, and various other signs and symptoms triggered by autoimmune illness, such as lupus, inflammatory digestive tract condition (IBD), celiac condition, and rheumatoid joint inflammation.

Many individuals that have actualy complied with the AIP

diet regimen record renovations in the method they really feel, along with reductions alike signs and symptoms of autoimmune problems, such as exhaustion and digestive tract or joint discomfort. Yet, while research study on this diet regimen is guaranteeing, it is additionally restricted.

This article uses an extensive review of the AIP diet regimen, consisting of the scientific research behind it, along with what is presently understood about its capability to minimize signs and symptoms of autoimmune problems.

What is the Autoimmune Protocol Diet plan?

A healthy and balanced body immune system is developed to generate antibodies that assault international or damaging cells in your body.

Nonetheless, in people with autoimmune problems, the body immune system has the tendency to generate antibodies that, instead of deal with infections, assault healthy and balanced cells and cells.

This can possibly cause a series of signs and symptoms, consisting of joint discomfort, exhaustion, stomach discomfort, looseness of the bowels, mind haze, and cells and nerve damages.

A few examples of autoimmune disorders consist of rheumatoid joint inflammation, lupus, IBD, type 1 diabetic issues, and psoriasis.

Autoimmune illness are believed to be triggered by a selection of variables, consisting of hereditary propensity, infection, stress, inflammation, and medicine use.

Additionally, some research study recommends that, in at risk people, damages to the digestive tract obstacle can possibly result in boosted intestinal tract permeability, additionally called "dripping digestive tract," which could activate the advancement of specific autoimmune illness.

Specific foods are thought to perhaps boost the gut's permeability, consequently raising your chance of dripping digestive tract.

The AIP diet regimen concentrates on getting rid of these foods and changing them with health-promoting, nutrient-dense foods that are idea to aid recover the digestive tract, and eventually, minimize swelling and signs and symptoms of autoimmune illness.

It additionally gets rid of specific active ingredients like gluten, which could create unusual immune actions in at risk people.

While specialists think that a leaking digestive tract could be a possible description for the swelling seasoned by people with autoimmune problems, they caution that the existing research study makes it difficult to validate a cause-and-effect connection in between both.

As a result, more research study is required previously solid final thoughts can possibly be made.

SUMMARY

The Autoimmune Method (AIP) diet regimen is supposed to minimize swelling, discomfort, and various other signs and symptoms seasoned by people with autoimmune problems by recovery their dripping digestive tract and eliminating possibly bothersome active ingredients from their diet regimen.

How does it work?

The AIP diet regimen looks like the paleo diet regimen, both in the sorts of foods enabled and stayed clear of, along with in the stages that consist of it. As a result of their resemblances, lots of think about the AIP diet regimen an expansion of the paleo diet regimen — however AIP could be viewed as a stricter variation of it.

The AIP diet regimen contains 2 primary stages.

The elimination phase

The initially stage is an removal stage that includes the elimination of foods and medicines thought to create digestive tract swelling, imbalances in between degrees of excellent and poor microorganisms in the digestive tract, or an immune feedback.

Throughout this stage, foods like grains, legumes, nuts, seeds, nightshade veggies, eggs, and milk are totally stayed clear of.

Cigarette, alcohol, coffee, oils, food ingredients, improved and refined sugars, and specific medicines, such as non-steroidal anti-inflammatory medications (NSAIDs) ought to additionally be stayed clear of.

Instances of NSAIDs consist of ibuprofen, naproxen, diclofenac, and high dosage pain killers.

On the various other hand, this stage motivates the usage of fresh, nutrient-dense foods, minimally refined meat, fermented foods, and bone brew.

It additionally stresses the enhancement of way of life variables, such as tension, rest, and exercise.

The size of the removal stage of the diet regimen differs, as it is generally preserved up till an individual really feels a recognizable decrease in signs and symptoms. Generally, many people preserve this stage for 30-90 days, however some could observe renovations as very early as within the initially 3 weeks.

The reintroduction phase

When a quantifiable enhancement in signs and symptoms and general health happens, the reintroduction stage can possibly start. Throughout this stage, the stayed clear of foods are progressively reestablished into the diet regimen, individually, based upon the person's resistance.

The objective of this stage is to determine which foods add to a person's signs and symptoms and reintroduce all foods that do not create any type of signs and symptoms while proceeding to prevent those that do. This permits the best nutritional range an individual can possibly endure.

Throughout this stage, foods ought to be reestablished individually, enabling a duration of 5-7 days previously reintroducing a various food. This permits an individual sufficient time to observe if any one of their signs and symptoms reappear previously proceeding the reintroduction procedure.

Foods that are well tolerated can possibly be included back into the diet regimen, while those that activate signs and symptoms ought to remain to be stayed clear of. Remember that the food resistance could alter gradually.

Therefore, you could possibly intend to duplicate the reintroduction examination for foods that originally fell short the examination every now and then.

Step-by-step reintroduction protocol

Here is a detailed method to reintroducing foods that were stayed clear of throughout the removal stage of the AIP diet regimen.

Step 1. Choose one food to reintroduce. Strategy to take in this food a couple of times daily on the screening day, after that prevent it totally for 5-6 days.

Step 2. Consume a percentage, such as 1 tsp of the food, and delay 15 mins to see if you have actually a response.

Step 3. If you experience any type of signs and symptoms, finish the examination and prevent this food. If you have actually no signs and symptoms, consume a somewhat bigger section, such as 1 1/2 tablespoons, of the very same food and check how you understanding of 2-3 hrs.

Step 4. If you experience any type of signs and symptoms over this duration, finish the examination and prevent this food. If no signs and symptoms take place, consume a regular section of the very same food and prevent it for 5-6 days without reintroducing other foods.

Step 5. If you experience no signs and symptoms for 5-6 days, you could possibly reincorporate the evaluated food into your diet regimen, and duplicate this 5-step reintroduction procedure with a brand-new food.

It is finest to prevent reintroducing foods under scenarios that have the tendency to boost swelling and make it hard to translate outcomes. These consist of throughout an infection, complying with an inadequate night's rest, when sensation abnormally worried, or complying with a laborious exercise.

Furthermore, it is in some cases suggested to reintroduce foods in a certain purchase. For instance, when reintroducing milk, pick milk items with the most affordable lactose focus to reintroduce initially, such as ghee or fermented milk items.

SUMMARY

The AIP diet regimen initially gets rid of any type of foods that could activate signs and symptoms for a couple of weeks. Each is after that reestablished independently to ensure that just those that do not activate signs and symptoms can possibly eventually be included back into the diet regimen.

Foods to eat and avoid

The AIP diet regimen has actually stringent suggestions relating to which foods to consume or prevent throughout its removal stage.

Foods to avoid

Grains: rice, wheat, oats, barley, rye, and so on., along with foods stemmed from them, such as pasta, bread, and morning meal cereals

Legumes: lentils, beans, peas, peanuts, and so on., along with foods stemmed from them, such as tofu, tempeh, simulated meats, or peanut butter

Nightshade veggies: eggplants, peppers, potatoes, tomatoes,

tomatillos, and so on., along with seasonings stemmed from nightshade veggies, such as paprika

Eggs: whole eggs, egg whites, or foods including these active ingredients

Milk: cow's, goat's, or sheep's milk, along with foods stemmed from these milks, such as lotion, cheese, butter, or ghee; dairy-based healthy protein powders or various other supplements ought to additionally be stayed clear of

Nuts and seeds: all nuts and seeds and foods stemmed from

them, such as flours, butter, or oils; additionally consists of cocoa and seed-based seasonings, such as coriander, cumin, anise, fennel, fenugreek, mustard, and nutmeg

Specific drinks: alcohol and coffee

Refined veggie oils: canola, rapeseed, corn, cottonseed, hand bit, safflower, soybean, or sunflower oils

Improved or refined sugars: walking stick or beet sugar, corn syrup, brownish rice syrup, and barley malt syrup; additionally consists of sugary foods, soft drink, sweet, icy treats, and delicious chocolate, which could consist of these active ingredients

Food ingredients and man-made sweeteners: trans fats, food colorings, emulsifiers, and thickeners, along with man-made sweeteners, such as stevia, mannitol, and xylitol

Some AIP procedures additional advise preventing all fruit — both fresh or dried out — throughout the removal stage. Others enable the incorporation of 10-40 grams of fructose daily, which total up to about 1-2 sections of fruit daily.

Although not defined in all AIP procedures, some additionally recommend preventing algae, such as spirulina or chlorella, throughout the removal stage, as this kind of sea veggie could additionally promote an immune feedback.

Foods to consume

Veggies: a selection of veggies with the exception of nightshade veggies and algae, which ought to be stayed clear of

Fresh fruit: a selection of fresh fruit, in small amounts

Tubers: pleasant potatoes, taro, yams, along with Jerusalem or Chinese artichokes

Minimally refined meat: wild video game, fish, fish and shellfish, body organ meat, and poultry; meats ought to be wild, grass-fed or pasture-raised, whenever feasible

Fermented, probiotic-rich foods: nondairy-based fermented food, such as kombucha, kimchi, sauerkraut, pickles, and coconut kefir; probiotic supplements could additionally be taken in

Minimally refined veggie oils: olive oil, avocado oil, or coconut oil

Natural herbs as well as flavors: as lengthy as they're not originated from a seed

Vinegars: balsamic, apple cider, as well as red red white a glass of wine vinegar, as lengthy as they're without included sugars

All-natural sweeteners: maple syrup as well as honey, in small amounts

Particular teas: green as well as black tea at ordinary consumptions of as much as 3-4 mugs each day

Bone brew

Regardless of being permitted, some procedures more advise that you modest your consumption of salt, filled as well as omega-6 fats, all-natural sugars, such as honey or maple syrup, in addition to coconut-based foods.

Relying on the AIP method available, little quantities of fruit could additionally be permitted. This generally total up to an optimum consumption of 10-40 grams of fructose each day, or the equal of concerning 1-2 sections of fresh fruit.

Some procedures more recommend moderating your consumption of high glycemic vegetables and fruits, consisting of dried out fruit, pleasant potatoes, as well as plantain.

The glycemic index (GI) is a system made use of to rate foods on a range of 0 to 100, based upon just what does it cost? they'll enhance blood glucose degrees, compared to white bread. High glycemic vegetables and fruits are those rated 70 or over on the GI range.

SUMMARY

The AIP diet plan generally contains minimally refined, nutrient-dense foods. The details over define which foods to consume or prevent throughout the removal stage of the AIP diet plan.

Does the AIP diet plan operate?

However study on the AIP diet plan is restricted, some proof recommends that it could lower swelling as well as signs of particular autoimmune conditions.

Could assistance recover a dripping digestive tract

People with autoimmune conditions frequently have actually a dripping digestive tract, as well as professionals think there could be a web link in between the swelling they experience as well as the permeability of their digestive tract.

A healthy and balanced digestive tract generally has a reduced permeability. This permits it to serve as an excellent obstacle as well as avoid food as well as squander continues to be from dripping into the blood stream.

Nonetheless, an extremely permeable or dripping digestive tract permits international fragments to crossover into the blood stream, then, potentially triggering swelling.

In identical, there is expanding proof that the foods you

consume can possibly affect your gut's resistance as well as work, as well as sometimes, potentially also lower the level of swelling you experience.

One hypothesis delighted by scientists is that by assisting recover dripping digestive tract, the AIP diet plan could help in reducing the level of swelling an individual experiences.

Although clinical proof is presently restricted, a handful of research researches recommends that the AIP diet plan could help in reducing swelling or signs brought on by it, at the very least amongst a subset of individuals with particular autoimmune problems.

Nonetheless, more study is should especially recognize the precise means where the AIP diet plan could assistance, in addition to the accurate conditions under which it could do so.

Could lower swelling as well as signs of some autoimmune problems

To this day, the AIP diet plan was examined in a little team of individuals as well as generated apparently favorable outcomes.

For example, in a current 11-week research in 15 people with IBD on an AIP diet plan, individuals reported experiencing substantially less IBD-related signs by completion of the research. Nonetheless, no substantial adjustments in pens of swelling were observed.

Likewise, a little research had actually people with IBD adhere to the AIP diet plan for 11 weeks. Individuals reported substantial renovations in digestive tract regularity, tension, as well as the capability to do recreation or sporting activity tasks as very early as 3 weeks into the research.

In another research, 16 ladies with Hashimoto's thyroiditis, an autoimmune problem impacting the thyroid gland, complied with the AIP diet plan for 10 weeks.

By completion of the research, swelling as well as disease-related signs lowered by 29% as well as 68%, specifically.

Individuals additionally reported substantial renovations in their lifestyle, regardless of there being no substantial distinctions in their steps of thyroid work.

Although guaranteeing, research researches stay little as well as couple of. Additionally, to this day, they have actually just been carried out on a little subset of individuals with autoimmune problems. Consequently, more study is required previously solid final thoughts can possibly be made.

SUMMARY

The AIP diet plan could help in reducing digestive tract permeability as well as swelling in people with autoimmune conditions. Little research researches record useful results in people with IBD as well as Hashimoto's thyroiditis, however more study is should validate these advantages.

Feasible disadvantages

The AIP diet plan is taken into consideration an removal diet plan, that makes it extremely limiting as well as possibly tough to adhere to for some, particularly in its removal stage.

The removal stage of this diet plan can possibly additionally make it tough for people to consume in social circumstances, such as at a dining establishment or friend's home, raising the threat of social seclusion.

It is additionally essential to keep in mind that there is no warranty that this diet plan will certainly lower swelling or disease-related signs in all people with autoimmune problems.

Nonetheless, those that experience a decrease in signs adhering to this diet plan could be reserved to development to the reintroduction stage, for worry it could bring the signs back.

This might ended up being troublesome, as continuing to be in the removal stage can possibly make it tough to fulfill your everyday nutrition demands. Consequently, continuing to be in this stage for also lengthy could enhance your threat of creating nutrition shortages, in addition to inadequate wellness with time.

This is why the reintroduction stage is essential as well as must not be skipped.

If you are experiencing troubles getting going with the reintroduction stage, think about getting to bent on a signed up dietitian or various other physician well-informed concerning the AIP diet plan for customized support.

SUMMARY

The AIP diet plan could not benefit every person, as well as its removal stage is extremely limiting. This can possibly make this diet plan separating as well as tough to adhere to. It could additionally bring about a high threat of nutrition shortages if its reintroduction stage is prevented for also lengthy.

Must you attempt it?

The AIP diet plan is created to provide help lower swelling, discomfort, or various other signs brought on by autoimmune conditions. Therefore, it could operate greatest for people with autoimmune conditions, such as lupus, IBD, celiac illness, or rheumatoid joint inflammation.

Autoimmune conditions can not be healed, however their signs could be handled. The AIP diet plan objectives to provide help you do so by assisting you determine which foods could be triggering your particular signs.

Proof relating to the effectiveness of this diet plan is presently restricted to people with IBD as well as Hashimoto's illness.

Nonetheless, centered en route where this diet plan is thought to work, people with various other autoimmune conditions could gain from it, also.

There are presently couple of disadvantages to providing this diet plan a shot, particularly when carried out under the guidance of a dietitian or various other physician.

Looking for expert support before providing the AIP diet plan a shot will certainly assistance you much far better identify which foods could be triggering your particular signs, in addition to make sure that you continuously fulfill your nutrition demands as greatest as feasible throughout all stages of this diet plan.

SUMMARY

The AIP diet plan could lower the extent of signs related to numerous autoimmune conditions. Nonetheless, it could be tough to execute by yourself, which is why support from a dietitian or physician is highly advised.

The profits

The AIP diet plan is an removal diet plan created to provide help lower swelling or various other signs brought on by autoimmune problems.

It is consisted of 2 stages created to provide help you determine as well as inevitably prevent the foods that could set off swelling as well as disease-specific signs. Study on its effectiveness is restricted however shows up guaranteeing.

As a result of its restricted disadvantages, people with autoimmune problems usually have actually little bit to shed by providing it a shot. Nonetheless, it is most likely greatest to look for support from a certified wellness expert to make sure you continuously fulfill your nutrition demands throughout all stages of this diet plan.

CHAPTER 2

The Wahls Diet plan for Autoimmune Disorders: 5 Tasty Recipes

We likewise consisted of Wahls' many preferred treat.

Nourishment plays an important function in enhancing our health and wellness. As well as if you deal with numerous sclerosis (MS), you recognize all as well well how vital diet plan remains in taking care of the signs and symptoms that feature this autoimmune illness.

The Wahls Method diet plan is a favored amongst the MS neighborhood, as well as it is simple to see why. Produced by Terry Wahls, MD, this technique concentrates on the function food plays in the monitoring of MS signs and symptoms.

After her MS medical diagnosis in 2000, Wahls chose to do a deep dive into the research study about food as well as the function it plays in autoimmune illness. What she uncovered is that a nutrient-rich paleo diet plan — high in vitamins, minerals, anti-oxidants, as well as crucial fat — assisted lower her signs and symptoms.

The Wahls Method varies from the paleo diet plan in one means: It requires more fruits as well as veggies.

If you choose to attempt the Wahls Method, you will appreciate a lot of spinach, kale, cabbage, mushrooms, onions, broccoli, carrots, as well as beets. You will likewise indulge on color-rich fruits such as blueberries, blackberries, as well as strawberries as well as grass-fed meats as well as wild fish.

Right below are 5 dishes to obtain you began on the WahlsMethod.

1. Rainbow Chard with Bone Brew as well as Bacon

This nutrient-dense Wahls-friendly dish from Phoenix metro Helix, a blog site produced by Eileen Laird for individuals complying with the autoimmune method (AIP) diet plan, is loaded loaded with micronutrients to assist assistance your health and wellness. The bone brew as well as chard provide crucial nutrients while the bacon provides this dish its scrumptious taste.

2. Poultry Liver Deep-fried "Rice"

Another Wahls-friendly preferred from the Phoenix metro Helix blog site is this dish for poultry liver deep-fried "rice." Made like a stir-fry, this dish teems with veggies like carrots, cauliflower, as well as scallions. Bonus, it is high in healthy protein.

The poultry liver materials you with high degrees of vitamin A as well as B as well as the dish consists of coconut oil, a prominent active ingredient in dishes for autoimmune illness.

3. Sluggish Cooker Spaghetti Squash

This dish from "The Wahls Method Food preparation for Life" will certainly please any type of pasta enthusiast. Spaghetti squash are a tasty as well as oddly pasta-like veggie that one could leading with all sort of scrumptious sauces.

If you utilize a sluggish cooker, you do not need to duke it out attempting to reduced the squash in fifty percent. Simply plop the entire point in your sluggish cooker as well as establish a timer. Roasting in the stove is likewise simple as soon as you halve the squash. You can surely roast or utilize your sluggish cooker to prepare all winter season squash, such as butternut, acorn, as well as delicata.

Offers: 4

Components

1 tool spaghetti squash

1 tbsp. ghee, thawed

1/4 mug dietary yeast

Sea salt as well as newly ground black pepper

Instructions

In a sluggish cooker: Place the spaghetti squash in the sluggish cooker, cover, as well as prepare on reduced for 8 to 10 hrs, or up till the squash really feels soft. Get rid of the squash as well as allow it awesome up till you can surely deal with it. Reduced in fifty percent lengthwise, inside story out the seeds, as well as scratch out the hairs with a fork.

In a stove: Preheat the stove to 375°F. Reduced the squash in fifty percent lengthwise as well as inside story out the seeds. Place the halves cut-side down in a big roasting frying pan or on a rimmed cooking sheet. Roast for 40 mins, or up till you can surely conveniently puncture the squash with a fork. Utilize a fork to scratch out the hairs.

Place the spaghetti squash "noodles" in a big dish as well as drizzle with ghee.

Spray with the dietary yeast as well as sea salt as well as pepper to preference. You can surely likewise leading this with your preferred Bolognese or marinara sauce.

4. Turkey Tacos

This dish, extracted from "The Wahls Method Food preparation for Life," isn't really a common skillet dish. As opposed to preparing your environment-friendlies with the various other components, you utilize the environment-friendlies as a taco "covering."

Butter lettuce as well as Boston lettuce or various other environment-friendlies, such as fully grown curly kale or collard fallen leaves, operate well.

Offers: 4

Components

2 tbsp. ghee

1 pound ground turkey

3 mugs very finely sliced bell peppers

3 mugs very finely sliced onion

3 garlic cloves, minced

1 tbsp. taco seasoning

1/2 mug sliced fresh cilantro

Warm sauce, to preference

8 big lettuce, kale, or collard fallen leaves

Salsa as well as guacamole

Instructions

Warmth the ghee in a stockpot or big skillet over medium-high warmth. Include the turkey, bell peppers, onion, garlic, as well as taco seasoning. Prepare up till turkey is browned as well as the veggies are tender, 10 to 12 mins.

Offer the cilantro as well as warm sauce on the side, or mix them straight into the skillet.

Separate the taco dental filling amongst lettuce fallen leaves. Include salsa as well as guacamole.

Roll or fold as well as appreciate! You can surely likewise offer the dental filling on a bed of environment-friendlies as a taco salad.

Food preparation pointer: You do not have to include sprinkle or brew to the fat when you are food preparation the meat for this dish.

5. Wahls Fudge

This is just one of one of the most preferred dishes from the Wahls Method, so it likewise shows up in "The Wahls Method Food preparation for Life" — with an included variant for white fudge.

This fudge preferences like an indulgent, wonderful deal with yet it is a lot more nutritionally thick compared to sweet, events, or various other wonderful treats. It is calorically thick, so it is outstanding for those who are shedding way too much weight.

If you are attempting to drop weight, appreciate it moderately.

Offers: 20

Components

1 mug coconut oil

1 tool avocado, matched as well as peeled off

1 mug raisins

½ mug dried out unsweetened coconut

1 tsp. unsweetened cocoa powder

Instructions

Incorporate all components in a food cpu. Procedure up till smooth.

Push the blend into an 8 x 8-inch glass cooking recipe. Refrigerate or ice up for thirty minutes to company up the fudge. Reduced into 20 squares as well as appreciate.

Wahls mentions she generally shops fudge in the fridge so it remains company. The fudge maintains for concerning 3 days — however it is generally gone a lot much faster.

Mexican delicious chocolate variant: Include 1 tsp ground cinnamon.

All you should learn about the AIP diet regimen

The autoimmune procedure (AIP) diet regimen goals to decrease swelling and soothe various other signs and symptoms of autoimmune problems. What can possibly an individual consume on this diet regimen, and exists proof of any type of advantages?

An autoimmune illness creates the body immune system to strike and damages healthy and balanced cells or body organs accidentally.

Typical instances of this kind of illness consist of psoriasis, rheumatoid joint inflammation, and lupus.

An autoimmune illness can possibly create swelling, and

tiredness is an additional typical sign. Depending upon the problem, extra signs and symptoms could consist of discomfort, swelling, skin modifications, and a high temperature.

The AIP diet regimen could help in reducing swelling and various other signs and symptoms of autoimmune problems. Discover more concerning the diet regimen and its possible impacts listed below.

Ways to follow the AIP diet regimen

An individual on the AIP diet regimen can possibly consume a lot of veggies.

The AIP is an removal diet regimen, so it entails not consuming particular kinds of food for a number of weeks each time and thoroughly keeping in mind any type of impacts on wellness.

Researchers have actually defined the AIP diet regimen as an expansion of the paleo diet regimen. An individual typically consumes lean healthy proteins, veggies, fruits, nuts, and seeds.

The AIP diet regimen concentrates on foods abundant in vitamins and various other nutrients. An individual adhering to it will certainly not consume anything with included sugar or various other ingredients that can possibly activate an autoimmune feedback.

An individual ought to abide by the diet regimen purely for a couple of weeks, after that gradually reintroduce the removed foods and take cautious keep in mind of any type of response. A response, such as a rise in signs and symptoms, can possibly show that they ought to omit that food in the long-term.

Discover more concerning the paleo diet regimen and what it entails consuming.

Foods to eat

Restricted research study shows which particular foods the AIP diet regimen consists of. An individual adhering to the diet regimen could have the ability to consume:

any type of veggies, other than those from the nightshade family members

premium fish and shellfish that are abundant in omega-3 fat

fermented foods

lean meats and liver

little quantities of fruit

oils, such as olive, coconut, and avocado oils

Generally, the diet regimen concentrates on entire foods and those that don't include ingredients such as sugar.

Foods to avoid

There are a number of food teams to prevent when adhering to an AIP diet regimen.

Bit advice is customized to individuals with any type of particular autoimmune problem, yet a study in individuals with IBS advises staying clear of:

nightshades, such as tomatoes, potatoes, peppers, and eggplants grains

legumes

milk

some veggie oils

coffee

eggs

nuts and seeds

alcohol

food ingredients, such as fine-tuned or included sugars

Discover more concerning the various kinds of autoimmune illness right below.

Why the AIP diet?

The concept behind the AIP diet regimen is that staying clear of gut-irritating foods and consuming nutrient-rich ones will certainly decrease swelling.

One hypothesis concerning just how autoimmune problems start is called the leaking digestive tract concept. It mentions that if there's an issue with the microbial make-up of a person's digestive tract, ecological causes of swelling — such as toxic substances and infections — can possibly violation the digestive tract wall surface and accessibility various other components of the body.

Fans of this concept claim that consuming the correct foods could aid stop signs and symptoms of swelling, although lots of specialists are doubtful.

Lots of advocates of the leaking digestive tract concept think that the AIP diet regimen can possibly aid stop the body immune system from assaulting cells and decrease the signs and

symptoms of autoimmune
conditions.

Does it work?

Couple of scientific research
researches have actually checked
into the efficiency of the AIP diet
regimen — generally or as a way
of taking care of any type of
particular autoimmune illness.

In 2017, some researchers
discovered that getting rid of
particular foods as section of the
AIP diet regimen enhanced signs
and symptoms of inflammatory
digestive tract illness.

In a 2019 study, 17 women individuals matured 20-45 with Hashimoto's thyroiditis, another autoimmune illness, complied with the AIP diet regimen as section of a 10-week wellness mentoring program.

Examinations revealed no modifications, yet the individuals reported a decrease in signs and symptoms and a renovation in their lifestyle. The writers recommended that the AIP diet regimen, as section of a larger therapy program, might aid individuals with the problem.

Some clinical evidence recommends a web link in between digestive tract wellness and inflammatory illness. An expanding body of research study, for instance, shows that there could be a web link in between microbial development in the digestive tract and inflammatory and autoimmune conditions, such as Crohn's illness.

Various other studies recommend that the make-up of digestive tract microorganisms could activate immune and inflammatory responses in various other components of the body.

On top of that, researchers have actually kept in mind that swelling influences just how well the digestive tract wall surface operates which food allergic reactions can possibly make it more permeable. This might show a web link in between issues with the digestive tract wall surface and autoimmune conditions, and confirming it will certainly need more research researches.

Sustaining asserts that the AIP diet regimen can possibly decrease signs and symptoms of various other autoimmune conditions will certainly need more research study.

Takeaway

There's inadequate proof to verify that the AIP diet regimen can possibly decrease swelling or profit individuals with any type of autoimmune illness.

Nonetheless, some research study shows that particular foods might make signs and symptoms even worse. These consist of extremely refined foods and foods which contain unhealthful fats, included sugar, or included salt. Consuming less of these kinds of food is most likely to be healthy.

Any person beginning a rigorous removal diet regimen ought to make sure, as reducing out legumes, grains, and milk, for instance, can possibly result in dietary shortages.

Review any type of large nutritional transform with a physician, that could have the ability to advise extra sources and aid establish whether the diet regimen appropriates.

Can possibly supplements aid with swelling? Discover right below.

Q:

What is the distinction in between the anti-inflammatory diet regimen and the AIP diet regimen?

A:

The objective of both is to decrease swelling in the body.

Nonetheless, the AIP diet regimen goals to decrease and reduce signs and symptoms of autoimmune conditions. It entails getting rid of particular foods that can possibly aggravate the signs and symptoms of present autoimmune illness.

The anti-inflammatory diet regimen, on the other hand, goals to decrease general swelling in the body.

An individual might utilize the AIP diet regimen as an anti-inflammatory diet regimen.

Relied on Resource Solutions stand for the point of views of our clinical specialists. All articles is purely educational and ought to not be taken into consideration clinical suggestions.